Food
To The
Rescue

Food
To The
Rescue

In Just 5 Easy Steps

Introduce Your Family To Healthy Living For Life

Dr. Jennifer Shell D.C.

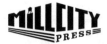

Mill City Press, Inc.
212 3rd Avenue North, Suite 290
Minneapolis, MN 55401
612.455.2294
www.millcitypublishing.com

This book is not intended to diagnose, treat, or cure any disease. This book does not take the place of seeking sound care by a qualified health care practitioner.

ISBN-13: 978-1-62652-054-7
LCCN: 2013903227

Cover Design and photography by Memory Laine Innovations

Printed in the United States of America

Table of Contents

Preface: Where You Learn a Little about My Story   **vii**

I.   *Introduction*   **1**

II.   *Step One ~ Know Your Definitions*   **9**

III.   *Step Two ~ Foods to Avoid*   **15**

IV.   *Step Three ~ Foods to Seek Out*   **29**

V.   *Step Four ~ How to Get the Good Stuff*   **39**

VI.   *Step Five ~ What to Do Once You've Got the Good Stuff*   **45**

VII.   *Reference Guide*   **53**

Bibliography   **61**

Preface

I had never dreamed of writing a book until I had my kids. My oldest son went to daycare for a couple of years. The facility provided breakfast, lunch, and snacks. My son rarely, if ever, ate any of them because I would pack all of his food. Breakfast at the center was traditional frozen waffles or the like. Lunch was canned spaghetti, canned veggies, and canned fruit. Snacks were always the fish-shaped crackers or teddy bear-shaped cookies.

No one knew this wasn't real food. It really started to bother me because no one else seemed alarmed. Then I realized people were being bamboozled. The government says these foods fulfill dietary requirements. Look at school lunches, for example: ketchup and French fries have counted as vegetable servings. It made me start to think about things. So I started reading. Then, on maternity leave with my second son, I started to write. People are starting to notice that the standard American diet isn't right. The blindfolds are coming off. Childhood obesity and diabetes are becoming topics of national conversation. People are starting to question whether the highly processed fats and sweeteners found in our most commonly eaten foods are safe. Change is in the air. I believe that if families educate themselves about food, we can change the industry.

I became a chiropractor because I wanted to help people heal naturally. As a chiropractor, I was very aware of how poor nutrition affects the spine and the nervous system. It's funny to me that most people really do not correlate their health to their lifestyle. So now I am on a mission to clear up all the nutritional misconceptions parents face. To help me do this, I utilize Nutrition Response Testing^{SM}, along with thousands of other practitioners. It is an alternative technique that addresses the body as a whole. I recommend diet modifications and very specific nutritional supplements to help patients rebuild their bodies from the inside out. Every day I help people relearn how to eat. I love nothing more than the look of shock patients give me when they feel better with food! They can't believe it's that simple. So many patients have been to multiple doctors with multiple problems that magically disappear when they nourish their bodies correctly. I want this realization for everyone out there looking for answers and searching for optimal health. I want my children to live healthy, happy, fulfilling lives. I want this for you and your children, as well. And you can have it. I see it every day. You have the answers right here. I hope you use them.

Chapter I
Introduction

The point of this labor of love is to teach you about food. You need to know the "real" right foods and the wrong foods so you can make informed decisions for your family. Teaching our children what foods are good and bad (and the reasons why) may save their lives. Good nutrition isn't hard. It doesn't have to cost a fortune. Unfortunately, when it comes to choosing what to eat, Americans are stuck in a rut. The media tells us what foods are tasty and good for us. Quick and cheap is the American motto nowadays. *We* should be the voice of reason for our families, *not* the manufacturers of processed foods. Author and researcher Michael Pollan points out that in 1960 Americans spent 18 percent of their income on food and 5 percent on health care. Fast forward to today, and we are spending 9 percent of our income on food and 17 percent on health care.[1] Additionally, more than 95 percent of our health care dollars is spent on disease treatment, and less than 5 percent is spent on prevention.[2] This shows that our priorities have changed. We don't take preventative measures. Instead, we eat cheap and get sick. Then we spend a fortune trying to heal ourselves once we get sick. What if we used food as our preventive medicine instead? We should be spending our money on eating well and taking high-quality supplements so we can enjoy our most valuable asset: health. Being healthy for as long as I can is my highest priority. What about you?

Processed food manufacturers have manipulated us all along. They are in it for the almighty dollar, not your beautiful little munchkin's health. "Experts suggest that until the age of eight or nine, kids aren't good at distinguishing the persuasive promotional efforts of advertisements from reality, nor are they adequately equipped to evaluate commercial claims."[3] We need to realize that advertisers already know this. Why do you think kids' meals come with toys? I don't put a new toy out for dinner. Do you? And this bribery works. "In a 2007 study, preschool children reported that food in McDonald's wrappers tasted better than the same food in plain wrappers, suggesting that branding can even trump sensory input."[2] What the heck? Commercials and advertisements convince our kids what to want and tell us what is good for our families, and we have trusted them. These foods being sold to us as fast, healthy, and easy are anything but beneficial in the long run. This is where the problem begins.

Look at the statistics. All of these diseases and problems are rampant in our country: diabetes, obesity, cancer, heart disease, ADD and ADHD, autism, anxiety, depression, chronic fatigue, and high blood pressure. Coincidentally, do you know what else is on the rise? Our consumption of sugar, chemically processed sweeteners, preservatives and additives, and hormone- and steroid-injected animal products. More than half of all Americans die of heart disease or cancer, and two-thirds are overweight.[4] These are diet-influenced conditions, yet we continue to eat junk and try to solve our diet-related health problems with drugs. And it's no longer taking until adulthood to catch up to us. "One in four children take prescription medication on a daily basis for chronic (long-term) illness."[2] One in four!

Essentially, the choice of what to feed our children comes down to us, the parents. Our kids will grow up with the same eating habits that we have. Monkey see; monkey do. Our nation is in trouble, and our kids need us. Currently, "only 2 percent of school age kids eat the recommended servings of all five major food groups."[2] So what are our children eating instead? Frosted cereals, pop tarts,processed chicken nuggets,frozen dinners,soda,supposed sports drinks and sugar laden fruit juices . We are raising the first generation that will not live longer than their parents because of obesity, diabetes, and heart disease. The Centers for Disease Control reported in February 2012 that 12.5 million kids age two to nineteen are obese in the United States. Sixty percent of overweight five- to ten-year olds show signs of cardiovascular disease.[5] I don't know about you, but that seems horribly wrong to me. We have to realize that what we eat has a direct effect on our health. If we eat poorly, our health is poor.

Drug commercials are obligated to disclose their known scrolling side effects. What if junk food companies were required to lay it on the line, too? What if, while you're watching the teenage boy slugging down an oh-so-re-freshing cola, a low monotone voice starts listing off warnings: "Stop ingesting if you begin to gain weight or develop diabetes, weak bones prone to fracture, or neurological symptoms or if you experience mood swings or trouble concentrating." That would be eye opening.

Our families need real food. Monosodium glutamate and red #3 don't count, folks! Sadly chemicals are everywhere in our environment. "Eighty percent of the toxins our children are exposed to come through the food and water they ingest. Our country uses fifteen trillion pounds a year of over eighty thousand different industrial chemicals, tested only by the manufacturers.[2] And thousands of different chemicals are used in our food! This means we are playing a possibly dangerous game without signing the roster. The more educated we become about what we eat, the better our decisions will be at the grocery store. Then we win. Checkmate.

🍎 Dr. Shells Tid Bit

Animals are usually fed grains that were sprayed with pesticides. Then the animals get injected with stimulants and growth hormones so the company can get them to the slaughter quicker. All of those chemicals end up in the meat we eat. Grains, fruit, and vegetables aren't exempt, either, unless they're grown organically. They are sprayed and many are genetically modified, which means their insides have been changed. Then a whole crop can be sprayed with pesticides so that the crop is the only thing left standing. These chemicals seep into every aspect of the foods that have been sprayed with herbicides, and then they go into our families' mouths.

I know it's daunting. You're thinking, "Lady, I don't have time for this! Between carpools, after-school commitments, and just trying to keep the house from drowning in clutter, I can barely get a shower in!" I know. I know. But it can be done, and it must be done. We can save our families from exhaustion, poor school performance, lack of concentration, depression, fatigue, mood swings, diabetes, heart disease, and obesity. But in order to do this, we have to change the way our households run. Not overnight, but slowly and steadily. Real food isn't tough to pull together. It just takes organization and commitment. Real food is what humans have always eaten until now. Once you decide to commit, for your family's health and the sake of their futures, you have to gradually make small changes. Sure, there will be times when it is challenging. Be patient, but don't give up and don't give in. Explain to your children why changing their diet is so important. Your family's future depends on it.

Here are some alarming facts. The number of preschool kids who are put on drugs for mood-related issues has tripled from a decade or so ago. The number of Ritalin prescriptions for *two* to *four* year olds has also tripled. Prescriptions for medications like Prozac have seen a tenfold increase for children younger than five.[5] Reading this made me want to throw up and cry because they are just babies. Let me mention that depression is not a "Prozac deficiency." I believe the majority of people see amazing improvements in their physical and mental health when they eat real food that nourishes their bodies. I see it happen daily. Once patients improve their diets, they constantly tell me how they've never felt better. They go see their medical doctors and find that they can get off their diabetes and hypertension medications. They lose weight, and their digestion is better. Their headaches are gone, and they are sleeping soundly. The list of positive improvements in my patients' bodies when they simply feed themselves with real, healthy food is truly astounding.

When we feel good, our confidence goes up, our mood is elevated, and our energy is better. Which parent do you want to be: short tempered, exhausted, and spacey or alert, involved, happy, and loving? Now, think about your kids. If you aren't giving them your all, they are getting the short end of the stick! Am I right? If you are energetic and happy, then you can help them succeed.

I love the analogy about crabs in a bucket. Did you know fishermen never have to worry about crabs climbing out of their buckets? If a crab tries to climb out, the other crabs will pull the "go-getter" down. Don't be a crab in a bucket by allowing your child to eat foods you know will prevent them from being their best. Instead, help push your kids to reach their potential! I always hear, "My kids won't eat blank-blank-blank." Well, we have rules in our house. If you don't eat the good stuff first, then there's nothing after it. Tough love isn't a mean thing here; I do it because I love my kids, just like you love yours. I am just saying be creative and persistent in helping them develop eating habits that will keep them healthy and strong. Don't be crabs in a bucket!

Lets take a minute and look at what we are up against. The soft drink industry spends roughly 600 million dollars a year telling us how we need their latest and greatest products.[6] Big time stars pimp processed and fast foods to your kids, and even athletes tell us how great this junk is. Companies are spending 150 times what they were about twenty-five years ago on marketing to kids.[7] If that isn't bad enough, here's what really gets me: this turns out to be about fifteen billion dollars a year targeting our kids.[7] That is a huge red laser target on our babies' backs. When is the last time you saw a cool commercial about fruits and vegetables? You're laughing right now because it sounds so lame! Imagine your kid in the grocery store begging you for carrots.

Carrots aren't frosted and they don't have characters on them, so it's a long shot! Family farmers and folks like you and me don't have that kind of advertising budget. So how can we fight back? We fight back by becoming educated. So, it's important to begin by learning the basics. We, the parents, must understand the good and the bad in foods so we can teach our kids. I don't want my kids growing up thinking frozen pizza rolls for dinner or donuts for breakfast are good choices. This is what they see and hear through all the media outlets. "Part of a complete breakfast." Yeah, right. Complete garbage. We have the power to educate our kids. Don't let the cute animal characters or the commercial mom tell your family what's nutritious. A cartoon and an actress are no substitute for your own educated guidance. So let's get educated.

Chapter II
Definitions

1. **Protein:** It is the fuel and building material our kids need to grow healthy muscles and minds. Kids need half a gram to a full gram of protein for every pound they weigh until eighteen years of age.[8] Adults need about one-half of our body weight in grams, if you're not overweight. If weight is an issue, scale it back a bit.

2. **Carbohydrates**:

   A. **Simple Carbohydrates:** These are foods that change into sugar. The body uses them for energy, but they burn up quickly, which leads to a fast drop in energy, mood, and focus. Our bodies store any extra as fat, so they are a big contributor to weight gain. They are to be avoided or limited as you become more comfortable with making menus.

   B. **Complex Carbohydrates**: These carbs break down into sugar much more slowly. This slow burn will lead to a steady mood, good focus, and energy. We have to have complex carbs to make energy. A good target is to get family members to eat in the range of sixty to one hundred carbohydrate grams a day. The better they get at this, the lower the number of carbohydrate grams should be. Approximately one hundred years ago, two-thirds of carbohydrates Americans ate came from complex sources like potatoes, vegetables, and whole grains (and that does not mean "whole grain" Wonder Bread, folks). The media tells us that we need lots of "whole grains" for a healthy diet. I believe this leads to way too many carbs and causes a lot of the problems that I listed in the last chapter. Today half of all carbohydrates are simple sugars. If you crave sugar or even complex carbs, you're probably not getting enough protein.[9]

Remember, your total grams of carbohydrates per day should be sixty to one hundred. That means carbs are gold because really this isn't very much. I admit, I can get a bit stingy about it. You have to think about what's important to you. I like to feel like I'm eating something valuable, which helps eliminate mindless eating. Think about the number of times when you have just stuffed your face with chips or cookies while say . . . cooking, talking on the phone, cleaning, reading, or playing with the kids. You get my point. Mindless eating.

3. **Fiber:** Fiber is a very important part of our diet. It cleans out gunk in your intestines and helps you go number two. If you don't go at least once a day, you are putting stress on your system because toxins aren't being eliminated. Low fiber intake is linked to many problems; the major one is cancer.[9] By the way, we need to get at least thirty grams of fiber per day. The average intake of fiber for the average American is 11.1 grams a day, while in China it is 33.3.[1] People, come on! I recommend you get most of your fiber intake from vegetables. At my office I make a big deal about constipation. Nobody likes to talk about it, but if your body isn't eliminating toxins, we have a big problem. Kids and adults need to move their bowels daily. It is the very first thing we address in my practice.

    A. **Insoluble fiber**: Moves all the crud through your bowels. I think of it like a toothbrush for your intestines.

    B. **Soluble fiber**: This kind of fiber helps level out sugar in your system. It can help you feel full longer too. I think of soluble fiber like a sponge, helping to suck up sugars so you don't get a huge sugar spike.

4. **Fats**:

    A. **Bad Fats**: Partially or fully hydrogenated fats are bad fats. They are also known as "trans fats." Look at the labels on salad dressings, sauces, and peanut butter. Bad fats are everywhere. They are dangerous.

B. **Good Fats**: Beneficial oils and essential fatty acids make up this group. These oils help protect our hearts from heart disease, and they help regulate blood pressure. They help fight inflammation, pain, and swelling. Also, good oils supercharge our kids' brains and make them smart. Mine are most definitely geniuses. (Okay, I may be partial.)

◁)) DR. Shells Tid Bit

Americans have fallen for the "low-fat" gimmick. But we need fats. Your brain can't work if it doesn't have fats. Low fat foods are typically higher in sugar, which is never good. To lose and maintain a healthy weight, we need to eat food with healthy fats included.

---

5. **Artificial sweeteners**: These are products made by chemicals that are intended to sweeten our food. The problem is that these products come with many known side effects and many possible side effects. That means the testing is inconclusive. Every one of these sweeteners is marketed as a sugar alternative that has low or no calories. Whether or not they have calories, they all perpetuate a taste for intense sweetness, which can turn into addictions to sugar and chemical sweeteners.[8]

> ### ◉ Dr. Shells Tid Bit
>
> Don't be fooled by "sugar-free" labeling. Food manufacturers just take out sugar and add a sugar-free alternative usually a chemical, cancer-causing sweetener.

6. **Preservatives/additives**: These are chemicals used to enhance flavor, sweetness, color, shelf life, and texture. You name it; there's a chemical for it. The problem is that many are linked to cancer and neurological problems. Artificial colors have been linked to behavior problems in kids. Clinically speaking, I see it all the time. My own son turns from Dr. Jekyll to Mr. Hyde with the flick of a gumdrop. Kids with autism, ADD, or ADHD can benefit a great deal from eating a diet free from artificial colors and preservatives. I have had children in my practice who struggle at school, and once preservatives are eliminated, they see a huge difference in their school performance.

Chapter III
Foods to Avoid

Why do we need to avoid the "food" that tastes so good and is so dang convenient? You know I have an answer!

1. **Simple Carbs**: As already explained in the definitions section, simple carbs are carbohydrates that turn into sugar in our bodies, giving us a quick burst of energy followed by a crash. It's known as the "roller coaster effect." These are the carbs that we get from most processed foods like white rice, corn chips, cookies, crackers, cereals, donuts, etc.

    A. **Wheat:** I know you may be shocked. We have been taught to believe that wheat is a staple in a wholesome grain diet. So why wheat? Most wheat is grown with pesticides, for one thing. You may say, "Well, I can get organic then." You can, but there's more. Mass production has led to wheat being harvested by big machines that are really rough. The outer shell of the wheat gets cracked during the process. Now air seeps into the seed and makes it rancid. Then during processing, manufacturers heat it up so hot it makes the wheat even more unrecognizable; it loses all of its nutrients through this process. Check out the whole process in Dr. Walter C.Willett's book, *Eat, Drink, and Be Healthy: The Harvard Medical School Guide to Healthy Eating* or read more about it on the Weston A. Price Foundation website (www. westonaprice.org). That's why that perfect, soft, spongy white bread is a true wonder. How can they call that bread?

B. **Corn**: You know how the Hulk had a genetic mutation that made him turn crazy (and green)? Maybe that's not so far-fetched! Corn seed is genetically modified to withstand bugs and disease. This is great for industry, but it's potentially not so great for our insides. Your genes are the fuse box of your body. If you flip the wrong switch, you may have a disease turn on. Genetic modification may mess with our wiring, and nobody knows what could happen. Unfortunately, food manufacturers have decided to push these potentially dangerous foods on us anyway. It's all about the almighty dollar. These foods save manufacturers money because they are cheap, so they don't want to look at the potential risks. We have to protect ourselves. So I read labels. If we don't buy it, they won't make big profits. It comes down to one of my husband's favorite sayings: "Grass roots, that's how we make change." (See, honey, I was listening.)

◉⁾ DR. Shells Tid Bit

Sweet corn that you eat off the cob is not typically genetically modified at this point in time. So that's good news for summer time cook-outs.

An important point to make is that sugar and corn sugar (also called "corn syrup") are not the same thing. Fructose coming from corn is metabolized differently than regular sugar and triggers the buildup of triglycerides (which is fat in the blood). High triglycerides can lead to heart disease, which, according to the American Heart Association, kills one of us every minute in the United States. On top of that, high-fructose corn syrup apparently doesn't trigger hormones that should tell the body it is full.[5] So we just keep eating and eating and eating. . . .

What's also alarming is that corn syrup and corn-starch, unless they are labeled as organic, are from genetically modified corn and are present in virtually all processed foods. These ingredients are in the dairy case, baked goods, the frozen foods section, and canned and boxed foods. You know what's coming, don't you? Yep, get rid of it.

2. **Bad Fats**: These oils are heated so that foods have a longer shelf life in the grocery store. The process destroys the good properties and makes dangerous ones that can develop into cancer, heart disease, premature aging, digestive issues, infertility, and autoimmune diseases.[10] Trans fats raise the bad cholesterol (or LDL) and lower the good cholesterol (or HDL). They also raise triglycerides (fat in a person's blood), which is the cause of all sorts of health problems. For example, researchers found that women with breast cancer had higher levels of trans fatty acids in their body fat than healthy women.[11] So think twice about that frozen dinner full of partially hydrogenated oils you pop in the microwave. Your ta-tas may depend on it!

    A. **Hydrogenated or partially hydrogenated oils**: These are also called "trans fats." These guys are a family of oils that have been constitutionally changed to make for a longer shelf life.

    B. **Margarine**: It is made of partially or fully hydrogenated oils. These oils are ironically not heart healthy at all.

    C. **Bad oils**: Oils to avoid are corn, soy, and canola because unless they are labeled organic, they are probably genetically engineered or modified. [12]

3. **Artificial Sweeteners**: Ah, sugar substitutes, marketed as the weight loss solution. Zero calories and you can still have all the sweets you want, right?

Sure, if you want to pay the price of the side effects. Saccharin (Sweet and Low), Aspartame (NutraSweet and Equal) and Sucralose (Splenda) can cause migraines, seizures, dizziness, vision problems, cancer, obesity, and diabetes, according to Kris Carr in *Crazy, Sexy Diet*. She also explains that sugar substitutes can cause obesity and diabetes. Isn't that ironic? The very conditions they are supposed to prevent or help manage are being caused by these substitutes. Sugar substitute consumption is reportedly linked to bipolar disease, depression, and panic attacks, not to mention birth defects, infertility, and miscarriage. Industry spokespeople argue that you would have to consume massive amounts of these sweeteners to experience bad side effects, but seriously, would you eat "just a little" rat poison? Speaking of rats, one study showed that rats fed diet sweeteners later consumed more calories, gained more weight, put on more body fat, and didn't make up for it by cutting back later.[2] Cut this out and tell your kids *why* they should too!

A. **Acesulfame K**: The FDA believes it may cause cancer. They aren't positive, but still they have decided it's okay to put it in gum, pop, and other stuff your kids love. The FDA apparently said that the tests on it fell short of their own standards.[13]

B. **Aspartame:** Also called Equal and NutraSweet. Aspartame is a possible cancer-causer, too. Joint pain may also be another adverse reaction from Aspartame consumption.[13] Aspartame breaks down into methanol, a common paint remover. What is even scarier is that methanol can spontaneously break down into formaldehyde (a chemical found in glues and adhesives). Double whammy! Methanol also increases dopamine in the brain and causes a high feeling, which makes it addictive.[13]

C.   **Sucralose (Splenda)**: Touted as a substitute made from real sugar (so it must be natural, wink-wink), Splenda is actually a sugar molecule plus a chlorine molecule. It's an organochloride, like DDT (an insecticide banned due to toxicity) or PVC (used in plastics and known to increase cancer and diabetes, to name a few risks). Mustard gas is another organochloride. That one is used for chemical warfare as a lethal respiratory poison.[13] So do we want to ingest an organochloride? No way, not even a speck.

D. **Saccharin (Sweet and Low)**: Saccharin has a long history of the government going back and forth on its safety. It is purportedly safe for humans, but ironically causes tumors in animals.[13] I don't believe our health is worth the unknown gamble. I would consider someone who knowingly licked a poisonous mushroom to be a fool. What about you?

4. **Preservatives**:

   A. **Monosodium Glutamate (MSG)**: MSG is in everything from salad dressing to frozen French fries and canned soup. It is used as a preservative to make food taste better. MSG is called an excitotoxin, which means it can literally excite nerve cells to death.[13] That is a very scary fact. Here's something even scarier: infants are four times more sensitive to excitotoxins than adults. So a pregnant woman or a mom who breast-feeds should avoid excitotoxins, such as MSG and Aspartame, like the plague. It can lead to brain damage.[13] Why, why, why aren't products containing MSG labeled "do not consume if pregnant or breast-feeding"?

   > 📢 DR. Shells Tid Bit
   >
   > MSG can also be found in "natural flavorings," and it can be called "autolyzed yeast" and "yeast extract," to name a couple of ways it's hidden in our food.

   B. **Sodium Nitrates/Nitrites**: These are highly carcinogenic (which means they cause cancer). They are found in most bacon, lunchmeat, ham, corned beef, smoked fish, or any other processed meat.

   C. **Sulfur Dioxide**: This destroys vitamin B1 and vitamin E. Vitamin B1 is important because it makes energy for our cells; every cell requires that. It is also needed to process carbohydrates, fats, and protein. Vitamin E has properties that may protect us from cancer and is important for good immune function overall. Watch for Sulfur Dioxide in dried fruits, soft drinks, and potato products.

D. **Artificial colors**: These include blue 1 and 2, red 3 and 40, and yellow 6. They are linked to behavioral problems. Must I say more?

E. **BHT & BHA**: These stop "food" from going rancid so it can stay "fresh" on your shelf for years in some cases. Ick. Dr. Benjamin F. Feingold, who wrote a book called *Why Your Child Is Hyperactive*, says that BHT can cause hyperactivity in children. These man-made chemicals are also potential cancer causers.

F. **Potassium bromate**: This is found in many bread products and also some soft drinks that are citrus flavored. It's bad news because they block the proper function of the thyroid.

5. **Soy**: Soy is marketed as a healthy food, but there is concern about its safety. Most of the soy used in the United States is genetically modified. For that reason I am very leary of most products with soy. Clinically, I find a lot of people to be sensitive to soy. Most infants I see cannot digest soy formula, and it leads to GERD (Gastro Esophageal Reflux Disease). Acid reflux is something very commonly seen in babies and kids these days. I have cared for many newborns that were put on drugs for acid reflux before they came to see me, which I find unbelievable. Babies (actually everyone) needs digestive juices to digest food; reflux

medications stop the production.[14] Also, soy-based baby formula is considered estrogenic, which can lead to increased estrogen activity and can lead to breast development in boys. Babies fed soy formula receive the equivalent of five birth control pills worth of estrogen a day. Soy can cause problems with the thyroid gland, hormonal imbalances, infertility, and immune system problems.[14] By impairing the thyroid gland, we get fat, our hair dries out (or falls out), and we become exhausted. What a pretty picture! I do want to mention that fermented soy like miso or tempeh are both fine, if they're organic. Fermentation removes the things that impair proper absorption.[14] Whole organic soybeans called edamame are acceptable as well. They are high in protein and fiber.

🍎) DR. Shells Tid Bit

Hidden soy can be in MSG, textured vegetable protein, mixed tocopherols, natural flavoring, and lecithin.

One company makes some soy protein shakes that I am ok with. Metagenics does rigorous testing on all of their raw materials and does third party testing as well. Their soy is non-genetically engineered and identity preserved so I find this acceptable if you are not sensitive to soy. I use many Metagenics products with my patients.

So my point is that most soy ingredients you see on packages in the grocery store are genetically modified. You won't know that it is or isn't unless it specifically says it isn't; and, odds are, it is. Read your labels! You're looking for a message that says "contains no GMO ingredients" or "certified organic." Certified organic foods do not allow genetic modification.

6. **Sugars**: Oh, my mouth waters just thinking about it. Just like an addict. Hello, my name is Jennifer Shell, and I am a recovering sugar addict. I admit it. If I have a little, then I need a little more, a little more, and it doesn't stop until I've eaten the whole cake. It is important for all of us to realize that sugar is addictive.[16] It also feeds disease. When I see a beautiful chocolaty treat, the only thing that holds me back is the thought of feeding a disease. A good example that illustrates how sugar feeds disease is a PET scan. Medical doctors use PET scans to look for cancer. They inject patients with a sugar solution and take a picture of their bones (like an x-ray). If that person does have cancer, they light up like a Christmas tree because the cancer goes right for the sugar. Cancer feeds off of the sugar solution like ants at a picnic. Bacteria, viruses, fungus, yeast, and parasites all love sugar. Sugar is actually an immunosuppressant, which means it shuts off the immune system for a period of time. That is like a bank turning off all its alarms and telling the robbers to come on in. It also causes mineral imbalances, which may not seem

like a big deal, but it's huge. For the body to digest one sugar molecule, it needs fifty-six molecules of magnesium. Magnesium is a crucial mineral because it plays a key role in bone formation, healthy muscle, nerve, and immune function, and it helps with healthy heart rhythm.[15] Without minerals available for the body to use in all of its processes, the body will have to pull them from tissues and bones.

📢 DR. Shells Tid Bit

In the United States, sugar production has increased from 8 million tons in 1900 to 115 million tons as of 2004.[13] That's a crazy huge increase! Funny how diseases of all sorts have increased exponentially, too.

To pull sugar from your family's diet will be tough, but so well worth their health. We use superhero and villain analogies at our house. If you eat sugar, then you turn into the "Joker" or the "Green Goblin," meaning you're crabby, mean, and nasty. "Superman" and "Batman" and all of your favorite heroes are so strong and smart because they eat their veggies and protein.

My beef with sugar is that it's in everything. Condiments, frozen foods, bacon, lunchmeat, and packaged products all contain added sugar. Start reading the labels and notice how often it is present in the ingredients list. You've got to be a savvy sugar detective. Manufacturers go to great lengths to make it hard to identify sugar in their ingredient lists. For instance, there is a new product called Promitor soluble corn fiber 70. It can be listed on labels as "soluble corn fiber," "corn syrup," or "corn syrup solids." It can also be labeled as "natural" on the label. Very sneaky. Corn syrup can be labeled as a fiber, and when people see "natural" they think "good for you." Another good tip is to look at the nutritional label under sugars. Four grams equals one teaspoon. A bottle of juice may say twenty-five grams of sugar, but if you look at the number of servings per container, there may be two or more servings in that bottle. That is fifty or more grams of sugar in one bottle of juice, which equals more than twelve teaspoons! Dump twelve teaspoons of sugar on your counter and try to eat all of it. Tell me that's not disgusting. That's just one juice. What about everything else you and your family eat that day? Ideally, a serving of food should have three grams of sugar or less per serving. It is virtually impossible to find numbers this low in packaged foods. Give your kid a juice box and a granola bar and you might as well be handing them a quarter cup of sugar—yikes! The average American actually consumes more than one hundred grams a day. The American Heart Association recommends that women consume not more than twenty grams of sugar a day. Men shouldn't consume more than thirty-six grams and children twelve grams. These values are *drastically* less than what most Americans consume. I want you to become aware of how prevalent it is so you can slowly wean it out.

Sugar alcohols are used so that products taste sweet with much less actual sugar. I am leery of them because they still cause addiction.[17] The more sweets you eat, the more sweets you seek. You will also get diarrhea and gas if you ingest too many sugar alcohols because they ferment in the gut. I do use xylitol in moderation. It is important to note that you should only use xylitol brands made from trees, not brands made from corn, due to possible genetic modification. Other common ones are mannitol (from seaweed), maltitol (from corn), isomalt (from beets), sorbitol (from corn syrup), erythritol (from a certain kind of yeast), and hydrogenated starch hydrolysate (from corn, potato, or wheat starch).

Chapter IV
Foods to Seek Out

1. Protein

    A. Meat/Poultry: Be aware that the USDA doesn't allow pigs, chickens, or turkeys to be injected with hormones, but they *are* allowed to be fed chemical growth enhancers.[2] Certified organic meat isn't allowed to contain any chemicals, so it's always the top choice. Farmers markets or local meat would also be good choices.

🔊 Dr. Shells Tid Bit

Free Range/Free Roaming: In order for meat or eggs to receive this label, the USDA says, "producers must demonstrate to the agency that the poultry has been allowed access to the outside." Unfortunately, this doesn't specify the amount of space outside or the time the animal spends outside.

Natural: No artificial ingredients or coloring was added.

Organic: The product must be at least 95 percent organic to carry the organic label. The product was grown, raised, or produced without the use of pesticides, insecticides, or herbicides.

B. **Fish/Seafood**: Seafood is a great source of protein, which is rich in omega fatty acids. Omegas are oils that are beneficial to our health. You can't eat fried fish sticks and think they count as a beneficial food because they are now nullified due to frying. Please just bake it. I would also avoid fish that may contain high levels of mercury, which is toxic. Shark, swordfish, and orange roughy are some examples. I also recommend that if you like canned tuna, you get cans labeled "troll and pole caught." This means that smaller fish are caught because they stay closer to the surface. The smaller fish hopefully contain less mercury. I find it at health food stores or online. It does cost more, so that is something to consider.

C. **Beans/Lentils (also called legumes)**: Legumes are great because they are high in protein and fiber. Legumes count as a complex carbohydrate, so they make a much better choice than noodles or bread. They are also cheap and easy. I soak beans and lentils in water overnight. This helps us digest them better, which also means you won't get as gassy from the little buggers. Another tip to help the bloat is to add a couple tablespoons of apple cider vinegar to a pot of soup about ten to twenty minutes before serving, don't worry, you won't notice any negative flavor. And your family will thank you.

D. **Nuts**: Avoid coated, honey roasted, or heavily salted nuts. Also, you may want to avoid peanuts and pistachios because they have been linked to high mold contents. Peanut butter should actually be avoided. Why, you ask? Peanuts go down a conveyer belt and the pretty ones get sorted into cocktail mixes. The ugly (a.k.a. moldy) ones go down to the end to be turned into peanut butter. The toxin on those moldy nuts is called aflatoxin. It is a huge cancer promoter. A test done on twenty-nine jars of peanut butter revealed up to three hundred times the amount deemed allowable in U.S foods.[1] I couldn't believe it either. We never hear about this in the news! Peanut butter is marketed as a kid staple. Do you know any kid who doesn't know what a peanut and butter jelly sandwich is?

E. **Seeds:** I love seeds because they are high in protein and are tasty. I recommend sprouted as the best choice because they are easier to digest. I buy them already sprouted and packaged when they go on sale at the health food store. They get pricy when you don't do it yourself. Sprouting basically involves soaking, you can easily find out how online. Isn't the internet so amazing?

F. **Eggs**: You can get "natural" or even "organic" eggs that are still coming from a chicken that never sees real light and is packed like a sardine in a hen house. I try to buy eggs that come from local farms or that say "pasture raised" because those chicks are where nature intended, roaming as they please. Eggs have good fatty acids and raise HDL, your good cholesterol—so don't shun them. Embrace that egg!

G. **Dairy**: I recommend raw dairy because all the enzymes are still intact. Unfortunately, it can be hard to find due to laws about pasteurization. Find a local chapter of the Weston Price Foundation on their website: www.westonaprice.org. They can get you in touch with local farmers who sell raw dairy. No other mammal drinks milk past infancy except humans. In my practice, I see pasteurized dairy linked to many allergies, digestive problems, asthma, ear infections, and eczema. However, if dairy doesn't cause you problems, cheese is a good protein, and it's low in sugar. It can constipate, so just be aware.

> **📢 Dr. Shells Tid Bit**
>
> Dr.Shells tid bit:<u>pasteurization</u>: heating beverages and food to specific temperatures for a certain amount of time to kill microorganisms. The con to this is that it kills beneficial enzymes that are naturally in things like milk to keep microorganisms from setting up shop.

H. **Protein Shakes**: Shakes are a staple at our house because they are fast and easy. We do shakes for breakfast, snacks, and even in the evening if anybody gets hungry after dinner. Good choices are whey, rice, hemp, egg, pea, and now even sprouted legume varieties. Please avoid shakes marketed for weight loss or kid protein shakes found at a traditional grocery store. The sugar-to-protein ratio in these shakes is alarming. I had a patient bring in a protein shake from a hospital where they were admitted that had nine grams of protein and thirty-six grams of sugar. This patient was diabetic. That is an alarming amount of sugar for a non-diabetic, not to mention a diabetic! So always read labels. The facts are all there.

2. **Complex Carbs**: This kind of carb has fiber and nutritional value that stick with you and give you fuel. I think it is best to get the majority of your carbs from vegetables, but you can do a bit of the list below. It's very important that kids get away from the over-abundant simple carbs constantly marketed to them.

Have you seen commercials for sugary breakfast cereals served with a banana and orange juice and the commercial says it's part of a complete breakfast? The whole "meal" is sugar, with not more than two grams of protein. How can this be considered complete? Complex carbs, on the other hand, will give your family some lasting energy.

📖 Dr. Shells Tid Bit

When reading labels, you can subtract fiber from the total carbohydrates to get the net carb value, which is part of your total allotted carbs for the day. So say there are thirty-six grams of carbs and there are six grams of fiber. Do the math, and you have thirty grams of net carbs.

A. Quinoa: It's a high-protein grain that cooks like rice and has a nutty quality.

B. Sprouted breads and pasta: These have more protein and live enzymes.

C. Sweet potatoes (and regular potatoes if you aren't trying to lose weight)

D. "All the veggies you can gimmie"

E. Squashes: acorn, butternut, spaghetti

F. Whole grains: Wild rice is a good choice.

A technical point that will come with time—when reading a label, look at sugar grams and carbohydrate grams. Avoid foods that have more than one-third of their total carbs coming from sugar.[9]

For example:

4g sugar   This is acceptable.

12g carbs

6g sugar   This is not.

12g carbs

I want to touch briefly on gluten-free carbohydrates. Gluten is a protein in some grains that people can be sensitive to. A severe case of sensitivity is called Celiac disease. To these people, such as myself, gluten is toxic. Symptoms can range from digestive problems like diarrhea to skin rashes, depression, and fatigue, to mention a few. The easiest way to see if you have a gluten sensitivity is to stop eating foods like regular breads, bagels, pastas, wheat cereals, muffins, crackers, and cereal bars for a few weeks. If you feel better during that time, than you may have a gluten sensitivity. Discuss this with your health practitioner to see if getting tested for Celiac disease is a good idea. Gluten-free baked goods and cereals are typically quite high in sugar and carbohydrates, so be careful and read labels if you choose to eat this way. Gluten-free carbohydrates are:

1. Rice
2. Millet
3. Quinoa
4. Amaranth
5. Buckwheat
6. Teff

3. **Good Fats:** Olive oil is very good for us, but never heat it! It is not stable at high heat, which means it goes rancid, which could potentially lead to cancer. Also, just an FYI: if weight is an issue, avoid too much olive oil. Its structure contributes to body fat, so don't overdo it.[18] I do all of my cooking with coconut oil or ghee. Ghee is also called "clarified butter." To make it, butter is heated and the top is skimmed off, just leaving healthy oils. Both are solid at room temperature. Coconut oil is high in saturated fats, which has traditionally given it the rep of being an artery clogger. But research now shows that coconut oil's saturated fats boost your metabolism, support the immune system, and actually improve heart health! So just scoop it out and heat it if you need a liquid. A beauty tip is that coconut oil is a great moisturizer. Just don't slip in the bathroom if you put it on your tootsies. Coconut has anti-fungal and anti-bacterial properties, too. I buy coconut butter and feed my kids a teaspoon here and there to boost their little immune systems. To aid weight loss, Mary Enig, a biochemist and pioneer in healthy fats and oils, recommends if you weigh 90 to 180 pounds, you take one tablespoon daily; if you are over 180 pounds, take two tablespoons. You can add it to hot tea or eat it plain. Do this for at least two months, and then slowly decrease the amount once you've lost the weight you didn't want.

🔊 Dr. Shells Tid Bit

Good fats are found in avocados, nuts, and seeds. I recommend some oils too. Just watch the cooking temperatures on each. For high heat cooking, use avocado oil. For medium high heat (425 degrees), use grapeseed or coconut oil. Don't heat flax or olive oil.

4. **Acceptable Sweeteners:** I have included in this section the sweeteners that should be limited, as well.

   a. **Stevia**: This wonderful leaf is actually thirty times sweeter than sugar, has negligible calories, and does not raise blood sugar—awesome, right? To use stevia powder in recipes, use one-half to one teaspoon in place of one cup of sugar and add one to two tablespoons of extra liquid. When you bake with it, don't expect the product to brown. I have cooked the crap out of stuff not realizing it was done! But, don't worry, friends. The "Is it done?" mystery is easily solved with the old-fashioned toothpick test.

   b. **Chicory**: The product Just Like Sugar is made from the chicory root.

   c. **Unsweetened apple sauce** (which would include the fiber) for baked goods

   d. **Unsweetened apple juice** (which does not have any fiber)

   e. **Date sugar:** It is full of vitamins, minerals and fiber.

   f. **Coconut sugar**: It is high in vitamins and minerals and does not cause a sugar spike, so I do like it in baking.

g. **Molasses**: It is extracted from sugar cane and also still has minerals intact.

h. **Pure maple syrup**: It has minerals like calcium, phosphorus, potassium, magnesium, and iron. Try to find organic, locally produced maple syrup because some producers use formaldehyde in their processing. Formaldehyde is a cancer causer.

i. **Raw honey**: It contains vitamins, minerals, enzymes, and antioxidants. Raw honey has beneficial enzymes that digest carbs. Remember, kids under one shouldn't eat honey because of a potential bacteria they cannot digest.

j. **Barley malt**: It has fiber, complex carbs, and potassium. Be careful if there is a gluten allergy in your family because barley malt contains gluten.

k. **Brown rice syrup**: It has complex carbs instead of simple carbs.

l. Limited amounts of sugar alcohols like Xylitol, etc.

****

THE BOTTOM LINE IS THAT SUGAR, ANY SUGAR, WILL FEED DISEASE. ANY SWEET TASTE WILL PERPETUATE THE NEED FOR MORE SWEET TASTES, SO THE KEY IS REDUCE, REDUCE, REDUCE!!!

****

Chapter V
How to Get the Good Stuff

First, while sitting and relaxing for the only peaceful two and a half minutes you get to yourself a day, make a list of breakfast, lunch, dinner, and snacks for the week. A mom I know, with six kids mind you, has a folder where she puts all her recipes for the week. She then goes through the recipes and writes down the ingredients she needs to get at the grocery store so everything is accounted for. She actually has a spreadsheet so every month she can rotate menus around. (I am not at all this organized, but we all need something to aspire to!) The point is, she doesn't run into a last minute panic, which could lead to a fast food dinner. With this plan in place, you won't either. Here is a sample grocery and menu list I would make to cover a week's worth of healthy eating:

- **For breakfasts:**
    - Eggs (to eat hard boiled, scrambled, in omelets, or whatever way you like)

- Turkey bacon (nitrate free) or sugar-free chicken sausage. I may mix into scrambled eggs if we are bored.

- Oatmeal (steel cut is best) or you can use quinoa flakes to make hot cereal, as well. No flavored oatmeal packets—loaded with sugar!

- Protein powder (I like sprouted legume, rice, pea, hemp, or whey proteins, but I don't recommend soy.)

- Unsweetened almond, rice, or coconut milk (to top "cereal" and for smoothies)

- Berries

- **For Lunches:**
  - Sprouted tortillas
  - Mayo
  - Hummus
  - Cucumbers
  - Carrots
  - Organic lunchmeat or at least nitrate free
  - Tuna fish
  - Lettuce
  - Lemon (I squeeze half of one over salad and pour on a bit of olive oil instead of dressing.)
  - Avocado

- **For Dinners:**
  - Peppers (to stuff with lentils and spaghetti sauce or ground turkey with quinoa, etc.)
  - Grilled chicken

- Homemade chicken nuggets
- Spaghetti with spaghetti squash would be the best. Sprouted grain noodles would be the second choice.
- Burgers (Try to go bun-less or put in a lettuce wrap.)
- Pot roast
- Steak
- Salmon
- Veggie burgers made out of lentils and quinoa
- Lentil soup
- Soup loaded with veggies (pureed if you need to hide them) with beans or animal protein

- **Snacks:**
  - Nuts
  - Carrots
  - Cucumbers
  - Snap peas
  - Jicama slices
  - Grape tomatoes
  - Sprouted pumpkin seeds
  - Sunflower seeds
  - Inchi seeds
  - Plain Greek yogurt with nuts, seeds, or berries
  - Raw cheese
  - Hard boiled eggs
  - Raw crackers made out of seeds
  - Sunflower butter

- ◆   Almond butter
- ◆   Guacamole
- ◆   Hummus

Now that you've made your list, let's talk about how to get the goods. Remember, ladies and gentlemen, plan ahead! Check online for any coupons you could use. Be sure you have eaten and aren't starving when you go to the store. You will fail if you go hungry, frazzled, and without a list. If the kids are with you, the same goes for them. The kids will be nutso, whining and pulling at you with the "I want ____" pouring compulsively from their sweet little addicted mouths. It makes me sweat a little bit just thinking about it. So have toys or snacks to keep them busy. They can help you, too. Give the little ones their own simple list with easy words or pictures from magazines like apples, carrots, or celery and make a game out of finding the items on their list. Stick to your list and avoid the center aisles as much as possible! That's the sand trap. All the processed foods are in those aisles. I'll admit it: I'm a coward. I cannot stare at the limitless rows of lovely, chocolaty cookies and not want them in my cart, so I don't even go down the cookie aisle! Fruits, veggies, meat, eggs, and dairy are all on the outside or outer aisles. You *will* need to venture into center aisles to get beans, seeds, nuts, quinoa etc., so go like hell and keep your blinders on!

Some people believe that eating healthier has to cost more, but you can do this on a tight budget. Seek out a local farmers market or a CSA near you. CSA stands for Community Supported Agriculture and is produce from local farmers. You typically pay for the season ahead of time and pick up a box of fresh veggies and or fruit weekly at a planned location. Local farmers provide fruits, veggies, dairy, meat, and, depending on where you live, maybe fish. The food is fresh and local, and the prices are good. There is no middleman. It's from the farm to you, directly. The selection of fruits and vegetables depends on your growing zone and the weather. Frozen veggies are a good alternative if cost is an issue. Please avoid canned produce because the cans leach BPA (a toxic plastic) into the food. They also have added sodium and sugar. Eden Organics is a very reputable company who uses BPA-free can liners. Look at what you are putting in your cart, read labels, and think about whether the ingredients will help or harm your family. Are the ingredients nourishing, are they harmful, or are the effects unknown? If we all start to spend our money on our health, we can start to change the industry. If we keep buying sugary processed foods, then that is what companies will keep offering.

When you get home, fruits and veggies need to be washed to remove pesticides, chemicals, germs, and other organic matter. There are many commercial fruit and veggie washes out there. You can also make your own produce wash if you are so inclined or on a tight budget.

Chapter VI
What to Do Once You've Got the Good Stuff

Now, what to do now that you have all the right stuff. Again, this takes planning. I try to prep on Sundays if I can. Set out storage containers so that as you wash and cut up carrots, cucumbers, peppers, snap peas, grape tomatoes, jicama, and celery, you can bag them right up! Do the same with your nuts and seeds. Little containers of guacamole, hummus, and nut or seed butters are good for dipping. Hard boil a bunch of eggs, maybe even peel them for easy access. Plan which meals will be served on which days so you don't have any last minute uncertainty. We always do the simplest meals on our late night or serve leftovers from the night before. Crockpot meals are also very convenient for busy evenings. If you don't do this planning ahead of time, you're doomed. You know after school it is go-go-go, and I don't want you to go-go-go to McDonald's for a quarter pounder.

How to transition a family of sugar addicts!

Picky eaters usually are not veggie lovers. They won't touch vegetables. Why are kids so picky? It's because they are addicted to sugar! Think about it. . . . Picky eaters love mac and cheese, peanut butter and jelly sandwiches, and noodles. Once addicted, we will all go to great lengths to get sugar and carbs. Ever gone on a late night convenience store run? I rest my case. Let's face facts. My son has grown up on veggies from the start, but he can still wig out and want more and more sweets if the sugar train has been rollin' through town.

The bottom line is to go slowly. Really, you don't have a choice unless you are ready for World War III at your house! Start to add in some good stuff before yanking all the sugar out. So give them a handful of almonds with that dessert and make a conscious effort to serve less dessert each time. At least some protein will help moderate the sugar spike so they don't totally tank. Each night, decrease the amount of dessert given and increase the amount of good stuff, such as nuts and fresh berries. These changes go for you and the kids! Once you get the bad stuff out, notice how moods change with certain foods. I have patients frequently tell me how good they feel when they eat better. If they eat something they used to now, they get sick. Their bodies are saying, "Heck no, you are not poisoning me!" Kids and adults need to realize that different foods affect how our bodies work and function.

Kathleen Des Maison, in *Little Sugar Addicts*, recommends going slowly and focusing on the process. The kids need to know your plan and why you're implementing it, and they need to know the process will happen step by step. Don't just yank everything out at once. You need time to implement the new changes; this is a lifestyle change, not a diet. Let the behavioral changes your child is making settle in. You have to commit to specific gradual changes and stick to your plan. Going slowly allows the neurological changes to settle in easier. It reduces the number of variables your kids are trying to deal with. You do not want anyone in the family to feel overwhelmed, you included. Remember the tortoise and the hare? Slow and steady wins the race.

If your kids will only eat carbs for breakfast (toast, waffles, bagels, muffins, cereals), start to move slowly into better choices. Instead of frosted flakes, serve Cheerios with Xylitol or raw honey. Try oatmeal with nuts, seeds, and fresh berries. I often try to make pancakes on the weekends. I use a gluten-free, sugar-free mix, to which I add ground flax and protein powder. Then I throw in blueberries, and nobody is the wiser! I make a lot of them and then freeze the extras. Then when we are in a rush, I pull out frozen pancakes for the kids and pop them in the toaster for a fast, pretty decent breakfast.

Heat frozen berries with some water and stevia for "fruit syrup." Try smoothies with protein powder, but call them "milk shakes."

For lunch, buy sprouted tortillas and make roll ups. If your kid will only eat jelly sandwiches, start to buy sugar-free nut or seed butters and low-sugar, natural jelly and slowly mix them in with the "regulars." If you are starting with traditional white bread, go to whole grain bread next and work your way to sprouted breads. While switching the breads over, start to serve less bread in general. If your kids are old enough to get it, explain that this isn't the best food for their bodies. It will not help them grow up big and strong, contrary to what advertisers or actors in commercials say. We are told that it is fortified with vitamins and minerals, though. What a line! These "nutrients" are synthetic (that means not from nature) and usually sprayed into the product, like an afterthought. "Oh hey, maybe we need to add some value to this Play-Doh, I mean bread."

Stage your dinner like a Broadway production in which all cast members are present as often as possible. Curtains please!

The show starts with the vegetable first. I tell the kids that they can't have more carbs, such as wild rice, until the protein and veggies are gone. My kids love carbs just like everybody else! My oldest son is five. He is constantly saying, "I don't like chili. I don't like zucchini," and on and on. My response is always the same.

"I understand, but I would like you to at least try it." I don't care what it is or how many times he has had it before. Usually he starts to eat it and then tells me how good it is. Insist that your kids try a new food, but don't force them to eat it if they aren't fans. Let them know they can try it another time. It can sometimes take ten tries before the critics say they like it, so don't give up on insisting that they try it. If they won't give it a try, don't sweat it. They will probably want to try it when they see you eating it regularly. Also, never tell your kids you don't like certain healthy foods. You might not be a fan of brussel sprouts, but who knows, maybe your kids will like them. Keep it positive. Remember earlier we discussed "monkey see; monkey do"? Kids are going to push the limits, and some kids are tougher than others. The show must go on. Keep yourself composed, and if you get frustrated, try not to show it. Every night the production will improve until, alas, a standing ovation.

Snacks will be a transition, too. If your kids eat donuts, pop, or candy after school, don't all of a sudden set out water and carrot sticks. You will get laughed at or screamed at. Neither is a pleasant reaction. Scale back and do this gradually. Make decisions with them about small changes they can confront. Tell them it is coming either way, so if they provide some ideas for the transition, it will be easier. Talk with your kids about better choices and how to incorporate them in their diets. You will most certainly hear things like, "I will die if you take this away from me!" (That would be the drama queen.) Or, "This isn't fair; you can't do this!" (The rebel.) My response would be that, as the parent, I have an obligation to keep my children safe, and I have learned that this so-called "food" is endangering their health. They may not believe you, or they may think you are overreacting. I wish that was the case! Get some of the books that I have listed in the back and let them read for themselves. Get some of the movies I have listed and have a family movie night. Explain that you like the way junk food tastes, too, but that doesn't mean it is good for us. It is loaded with chemicals that lure us in so we'll want it all the time. This makes companies very rich, while we get very fat, tired, and diseased. Ask them if they're cool with that. Some kids may say yes. Nobody said this would be easy, but you can't quit.

Slowly introduce more fresh vegetables and healthy proteins, and stop bringing sugar, simple carbs, and processed foods into your house. If you stop buying junk, at least they aren't getting it at home. The new good foods in the house need to be easy to access so they can snack on them when they are hungry; so make them readily available. It's more work for you, I know, but it's our job, really. Tough love can be a good thing. People, we are strong and fake food is weak, so please take the reigns. We can win, household by household.

I know I have repeated myself throughout this book. It was intentional. Sometimes it takes reading things many times over to make it stick. First, it has to stick on you; then you make it stick on your kids. I know you can do this. Commit to it. Here are a few key "take aways" to start with.

- To start, pick one thing to avoid and slowly eliminate it: wheat, corn, bad fats, artificial sweeteners, preservatives, soy, or sugar.

- Be patient and persistent.

- Plan! Plan! Plan!

- Educate the family as much as you can, tailored to their age and understanding.

- Read this book over and over until you know it like the back of your hand.

- Don't beat yourself up if you fall off the wagon. Dust yourself off and hop back on—there is work to be done!

Lastly, thank you for caring enough about yourself and your family to want to change and for seeing the need for change. I hope this book is helpful and the changes become real to you. We are the vehicles of change. Never diminish your power!

Chapter VII
Reference Guide

The following are lists of foods and their specific properties. This is intended to help you make better decisions by having examples to compare.

Carbohydrate grams in some simple carbs
1. White rice: 1 cup cooked has 44g carbs
2. Rice cake: 7g
3. Most breads: 12g carbs per slice
4. Pasta: 1 cup = 36–43g
5. Tortillas: corn and wheat varietiesvary from 5–13g
6. Muffin: most seem to be 30–50g
7. Bagel: 50–60g
8. Most cereals: 10–40g
9. Cake: 14–50g
10. Crackers: 10 crackers would have 10–30g
11. Pancake:10–12g
12. Waffle: 13–19g
13. Toaster-type pastries: 15–34g
14. Cookie: 3–19g
15. Donut: 12–34g
Notice the giant variants in carbohydrate grams. You must read the label.

SUGARS TO AVOID
High Fructose Corn Syrup
"White" Sugar
Powdered Sugar
Brown Sugar
Agave
LIMITED SUGARS
Fruit Sugars
Coconut Sugar
Molasses
Maple Syrup
Raw Honey
Barley Malt
Brown Rice Syrup
Sugar Alcohols
ACCEPTABLE SWEETENERS
Stevia
Chicory Root

MEATS: protein measured in 1oz. servings
1.   Turkey breast = 5g
2.   Pork = 7g
3.   Chicken = 8g
4.   Lamb = 6g
5.   Beef = 8g
6.   Venison = 8g
7.   Buffalo =6g
8.   Ostrich = 6g

SEAFOOD: all are about 6g of protein per oz.
1.   Salmon
2.   Shrimp
3.   Trout
4.   Scallops
5.   Cod
6.   Halibut
7.   Tuna (1 oz. = 8 grams of protein)

BEANS/LENTILS: protein measured in 1 cup servings
1.   Garbanzo beans(or chick peas) = 15 g
2.   Black eyed peas = 13 g
3.   Pinto beans = 14 g
4.   Black beans = 15 g
5.   Northern beans =19 g
6.   Kidney beans = 15 g
7.   Lentils = 18 g

NUTS: protein measured in 1oz. serving, best choice is raw sprouted.
1.   Almonds = 6g
2.   Pecans = 3g
3.   Brazil nuts = 4g
4.   Walnuts = 4g
5.   Macadamia nuts = 2g
6.   Peanuts = 7g
7.   Cashews = 5g
8.   Pistachios = 6g

SEEDS: protein measured in grams
1.   Sesame (when made into a spread it is called tahini)- 1oz = 5g
2.   Sunflower- 1oz. = 6 or 7 g
3.   Sunflower seed butter (watch out for sugar content)- 1 TBS= 3g
4.   Pumpkin (also called pepitos)- 1 oz. = 7 g
5.   Chia- 1 TBS= 3g
6.   Hemp- 3 TBS = 15 g
7.   Flax -2 TBS = 4 g (these need to be ground so that you can absorb all the nutrients)
8.   Inchi -1 oz.=8 g

Dairy: Consider raw—a one-ounce cube of cheese has about five grams of protein. Cottage cheese is a good choice, too. Four ounces of cottage cheese has about fourteen grams of protein. Greek yogurt is also good due to protein content. But, ah-ah-ah, not the fruity ones, mister! Eat plain with fresh fruit on top. Traditional fruit-sweetened yogurt has crazy amounts of sugar. Also, don't be fooled by "low-sugar" varieties. They use artificial sweeteners. Start by mixing a little Greek yogurt in with what the kids are used to. Then start to gradually transition it over to plain Greek yogurt and put different toppings on it. Let them sprinkle berries, nuts, or seeds and mix in a tiny bit of a healthy sweetener like stevia.

Some Websites To Get You Started

CCHR.org (citizens commission for human rights)

paleoparents.com

 elanaspantry.com

chocolatecoveredkatie.com

damyhealth.com

mercola.com

foodtotherescue.com

Movies to Check Out

Super Size Me
Two Angry Moms
Food, Inc.
Food Matters
King Corn
Ingredients
Forks Over Knives
The Gerson Miracle
The Beautiful Truth

Recommended Books

In addition to the books in the bibliography, please check out the following books:

Appleton, Nancy, and G. N. Jacobs. *Suicide by Sugar: A Startling Look at Our #1 National Addiction*. Garden City Park: Square One, 2009.

Davis, William. *Wheat Belly: Lose the Wheat, Lose the Weight, and Find Your Path Back to Health*. Emmaus: Rodale, 2011.

Dumke, Nicolette M. *Allergy Cooking with Ease*. Lancaster: Starburst, 1992.

Dumke, Nicolette M. *Allergy Cooking with Ease: The No Wheat, Milk, Eggs, Corn, Soy, Yeast, Sugar, Grain and Gluten Cookbook*. Louisville: Adapt, 2007.

Ettlinger, Steve. *Twinkie, Deconstructed: My Journey to Discover How the Ingredients Found in Processed Foods*

Are Grown, Mined (Yes, Mined), and Manipulated into What America Eats. New York: Hudson Street, 2007.

Fuhrman, Joel. *Eat to Live: The Amazing Nutrient-rich Program for Fast and Sustained Weight Loss*. New York: Little, Brown and Co., 2011.

Gates, Donna, and Linda Schatz. *The Body Ecology Diet: Recovering Your Health and Rebuilding Your Immunity*. Carlsbad: Hay House, 2011.

Gittleman, Ann Louise. *The Fat Flush Plan*. New York: McGraw-Hill, 2002.

Kirkland, James, and Tanya Kirkland. *Sugar-free Cooking with Stevia: The Naturally Sweet & Calorie-free Herb*. Arlington: Crystal Health Pub., 2000.

Martin, Jeanne Marie, and Zoltan P. Rona. *Complete Candida Yeast Guidebook: Everything You Need to Know about Prevention, Treatment, & Diet*. Roseville: Prima Health, 2000.

McCarthy, Jenny, and Jerry Kartzinel. *Healing and Preventing Autism: A Complete Guide*. New York: Plume, Penguin, 2010.

McMillan, Tracie. *The American Way of Eating: Undercover at Walmart, Applebee's, Farm Fields, and the Dinner Table*. New York: Scribner, 2012.

Mercola, Joseph, and Ben Lerner. *Generation XL: Raising Healthy, Intelligent Kids in a High-tech, Junk-food World*. Nashville: Thomas Nelson, 2007.

O'Brien, Robyn, and Rachel Kranz. *The Unhealthy Truth: How Our Food Is Making Us Sick and What We Can Do about It*. New York: Broadway, 2009.

O'Brien, Susan. *Gluten-free, Sugar-free Cooking: Over 200 Delicious Recipes to Help You Live a Healthier, Allergy-free Life*. New York: Marlowe & Co, 2006.

Pollan, Michael. *In Defense of Food: An Eater's Manifesto*. New York: Penguin, 2008.

Price, Weston A. *Nutrition and Physical Degeneration*. La Mesa: Price-Pottenger NutritionFoundation, 2009.

Severson, Kim, and Cindy Burke. *The Trans Fat Solution: Cooking and Shopping to Eliminate the Deadliest Fat from Your Diet*. Berkeley: Ten Speed, 2003.

Smith, Jeffrey M. *Seeds of Deception: Exposing Industry and Government Lies about the Safety of the Genetically Engineered Foods You're Eating*. Fairfield: Yes, 2003.

Taubes, Gary. *Why We Get Fat: And What to Do about It*. New York: Anchor, 2011.

Willett, Walter, P. J. Skerrett, Edward L. Giovannucci, and Maureen Callahan. *Eat, Drink, and Be Healthy: The Harvard Medical School Guide to Healthy Eating*. New York: Simon & Schuster Source, 2001.

Bibliography

1. Campbell, T. Colin, and Thomas M. Campbell. *The China Study: The Most Comprehensive Study of Nutrition Ever Conducted and the Startling Implications for Diet, Weight Loss and Long-term Health.* Dallas: BenBella, 2005.

2. Kalafa, Amy. *Lunch Wars: How to Start a School Food Revolution and Win the Battle for Our Children's Health.* New York: Jeremy P. Tacher/Penguin, 2011.

3. Jana, Laura A., and Jennifer Shu. *Food Fights: Winning the Nutritional Challenges of Parenthood Armed with Insight, Humor and a Bottle of Ketchup.* Washington, DC: American Academy of Pediatrics, 2008.

4. Carr, Kris. *Crazy Sexy Diet: Eat Your Veggies, Ignite Your Spark, and Live like You Mean It!* Guilford: Skirt!, 2011.

5. Sears, William. *The NDD Book: How Nutrition Deficit Disorder Affects Your Child's Learning, Behavior,*

and Health, and What You Can Do about It—without Drugs. New York: Little, Brown, 2009.

6. Critser, Greg. *Fat Land: How Americans Became the Fattest People in the World.* Boston, MA: Houghton Mifflin, 2003.

7. Bennett, Connie, and Stephen T. Sinatra. *Sugar Shock!: How Sweets and Simple Carbs Can Derail Your Life, and How You Can Get Back on Track.* New York: Berkley, 2007.

8. Bean, Anita. *Awesome Foods for Active Kids: The ABCs of Eating for Energy and Health.* Alameda: Hunter House, 2006.

9. Gittleman, Ann Louise. *Get the Sugar Out: 501 Simple Ways to Cut the Sugar out of Any Diet.* New York: Three Rivers, 2008.

10. Enig, Mary G., and Sally Fallon. *Eat Fat, Lose Fat: Lose Weight and Feel Great with Three Delicious, Science-based Coconut Diets.* New York: Hudson Street, 2005.

11. Buff, Sheila. *The Good Fat, Bad Fat Counter.* New York: St Martin's Paperbacks, 2002.

12. Enig, Mary G. *Know Your Fats: The Complete Primer for Understanding the Nutrition of Fats, Oils and Cholesterol.* Silver Spring: Bethesda, 2000.

13. Mercola, Joseph, and Kendra Degen. Pearsall-Nelson. *Sweet Deception: Why Splenda, Nutrasweet, and the FDA May Be Hazardous to Your Health.* Nashville: Nelson, 2006.

14. Brownstein, Dr. David. "Soy Good For You? Not So Fast." *Natural Way to Health* 4 (Nov. 2011): 1.

15. Campbell-McBride, Natasha. *Gut and Psychology Syndrome: Natural Treatment for Autism, Dyspraxia, A.D.D., Dyslexia, A.D.H.D., Depression, Schizophrenia.* Cambridge: Medinform, 2004.

16. DesMaisons, Kathleen. *Little Sugar Addicts: End the Mood Swings, Meltdowns, Tantrums, and Low Self-esteem in Your Child Today.* New York: Three Rivers, 2004.

17. Hunt, Douglas. *No More Cravings.* New York: Warner, 1987.

18. Fallon, Sally, Mary G. Enig, Kim Murray, and Marion Dearth. *Nourishing Traditions: The Cookbook that Challenges Politically Correct Nutrition and the Diet Dictocrats.* Washington, DC: NewTrends Pub., 2001.

19. Brownstein, David, and Sheryl Shenefelt. *The Guide to Healthy Eating.* Birmingham: Healthy Living, 2010.